BALANCED EPIPHANY

Harnessing the Inner You: CHAKRAS

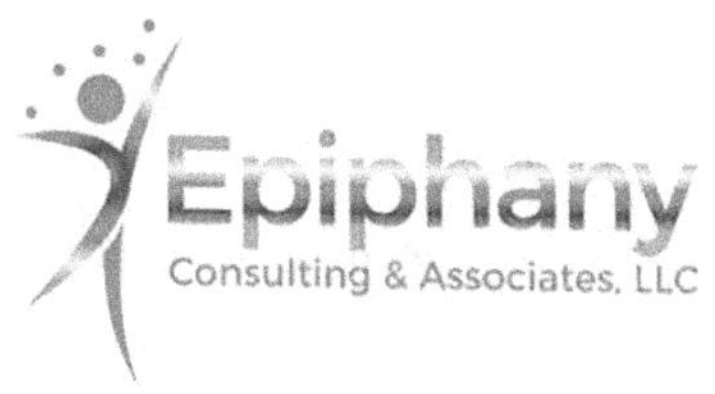

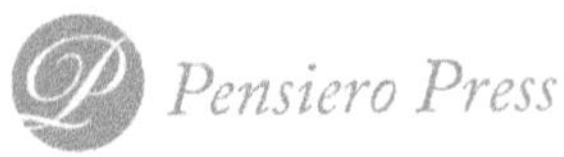

www.ThePensieroPress.com

Books are available through Pensiero Press at special discounts for bulk purchases for the purpose of sales promotion, seminar attendance, or educational purposes. Special volumes can be created for specific purposes and to organizational specifications. Please contact us for further details.

DR. TEMEAKA GRAY

Website: https://temeakagray.wixsite.com/epiphanyconsulting

Facebook

https://www.facebook.com/temeaka.gray
https://www.facebook.com/Epiphany-Health-Tips-289518337764385/
https://www.facebook.com/groups/217210798295890/

Twitter: @DocGrayCNP

ISBN: 978-1-7356817-7-1

Kindle and electronic versions available

Design & production: www.thebookcouple.com

Contents

This book is dedicated to life, love, and learning,
and to all those who are on a journey.

Foreword

Sheikess Temeaka Gray El, PsyD, MBA, MSN, APRN-BC

This is how most will be introduced to the author of this book; let me assure you she is infinitely more. Each interaction in the time that I've known this dynamic woman has bettered me.

In the times we live, the human family is seeking truth. This truth comes to us in many forms, usually in multiple forms of information. Dr. Gray El has taken these disparate and sometimes banal forms of data and reduced them to kernels of knowledge. This ability and talent are no doubt linked to her training. I request one thing of you as read this book. Read with your spirit, for that is how this work was prepared. One thing that some will not see beyond the letters behind Dr. Gray El's name is her deep spirituality and her desire to see humanity made whole. I want you to see this. Yes, she has studied the functions of body and mind; with this work she gives to the world deeper insights into your undying spirit.

After receiving a Reiki treatment from Dr. Gray El with over 120 miles between, you'll quickly understand the efficacy and implementation of her knowledge is at mastery level. I have had the humbling pleasure to converse and meet with world class energy healers around the globe, and place Dr. Gray El down as one of them. In my own pursuits of knowledge in healing, I've read no less than 30 books on chakras, chi, prana, and many other esoteric forms of working with nature. In a brief conversation about this book, Dr. Gray El gave me several new insights into how the chakras really work and how I can continue to grow in knowledge of them. Incredible!

Understanding there was never a time when man was not gives a greater awareness to the phrase there is nothing new under the sun (nor above it). As you prepare to not just read but experience Harmonic Balance, realize it is the synthesis of Dr. Temeaka Gray El's spirit, distilled by her mind, activated by the knowledge therein, encompassed by spirituality on a foundation of love.

Digest this book into the soul and increase in Love, Light, and Universal Peace for the unity of the human family.

Ase',
Salih Nurruddin Bey

Preface

Greetings! Throughout my life, I have looked inward. That is not to say that my introspection was always productive. More often than not, my introspection resulted in trying to figure out my part in something and ultimately accepting most, if not all, the blame for anything negative and little, if any, of the praise for anything positive. Despite this, my awkward feelings of not being enough and always being the cause of problems, I achieved what many deem success yet none of the so-called success made me happy.

I always planned to be a nurse (and a doctor), so, it was no surprise to family members and friends when I became a nurse, nurse practitioner, and then earned my doctorate in health and wellness psychology. What family did not know is that becoming a nurse, nurse practitioner, and earning a doctorate (in anything) was a surprise to me and none of the so-called success really fulfilled me. At one point, I began to explore spirituality, mostly the impact of spirituality of self-actualization. I have been very interested in the concept of self-actualization since I first learned about Maslow's Hierarchy of Needs in my freshman or sophomore year of college. I remember reading that most people never master self-actualization even if they master the four levels that came before it. This topic interested me but required that I step outside of the what I considered normal life and step into something that seemed somewhat scary, foreign, and strange. This path did not represent any specific religion or designated path other than one that I defined for myself in self-exploration and having grown up in a family that is passionate about religion; perhaps that was the scariest part of all.

In 2016, feelings of being unfulfilled with life began to tug at me so strongly that I knew that I had to do something. I needed to learn more about why I was feeling so unfulfilled. I began to explore my inner self and in late 2017, I began to investigate my true purpose. I was led to various types of healing practices. Ordinarily, seeing emails, informercials, and social media advertisements about healing practices would not have been a surprise because I always wanted to help people and I saw patients as a Nurse Practitioner. Par for the course, right? Except that this time, it was different. I felt different. This time I felt that I should be providing healing to more than just the patient who came to the office to see me for patient encounters. That epiphany led me to another exploration, one that I explored previously and let fall by the wayside. This journey into the metaphysical world of sacred geometry, personal energy, and self-improvement afforded the ability to create a more positive internal atmosphere for myself and is the drive behind sharing this information with all who are willing to listen. This book is the first of at least five books to share what I have learned with a deep-rooted desire that this information will assist others in reaching the same internal peace and positive environment for themselves.

Acknowledgments

A special thank you to the Universal Life Force, the source of all things including interconnectedness; the one who connects you and the one who connects me.

Introduction

Two types of energy are physical energy and subtle energy. Physical energy moves the physical body; whereas subtle energy is the vibrations that extend beyond the physical world. Three systems that make up subtle energetic anatomy are auric fields, meridians, and chakras. The subtle energetic anatomy system is responsible for regulating subtle energy (Dale, 2016).

Alchemy

Alchemy is a philosophical tradition practiced in Europe, Asia, and Africa during the Middle Age and Renaissance periods. Practitioners of Alchemy were known as *Alchemists.* The focus of alchemy was to purify and perfect objects. Alchemists commonly focused on transformation of base metals into noble metals, creation of an elixir for mortality, creation of a remedy that would cure any disease, and the development of a universal solvent that had the ability to dissolve everything. Modern discussions about alchemy focus on esoteric spiritual practices or exoteric practical applications. Alchemy is said to be the precursor of modern chemistry.

Sacred Geometry

Sacred geometry refers to patterns, designs, and structures found in nature. In this concept, the word *sacred* refers to being connected to the source of everything. The geometry of this concept is named sacred because the same geometric proportions, measurements, and ratios can be found everywhere. Hexahedron, icosahedron, tetrahedron, octahedron, dodecahedron, merkaba, and sphere are the platonic solid shapes of sacred geometry. Everything. including humans. are geometric at the core. Evidence of sacred geometry in humans is cellular structure, atomic structure, and Deoxyribonucleic Acid (DNA) (Lon, 2016). Sacred geometry is often used to make grids for crystal energy healing work and seen in the architecture of cathedrals and other holy buildings.

Quantum Field

The quantum field is a space of endless possibilities. The language of the soul, *sacred geometry*, allows us to access the quantum field because it is the language understood by the subconscious mind; the soul (Lon, 2016). Relaxing our conscious mind allows the ability to explore the endless possibilities available to us. The word *quantum* is not reserved for spiritual or metaphysical practices; quantum theory is a basis for physics and mechanics. In the world of energy healing and metaphysics, the quantum field is used as an area to assist with healing of symptoms. Quantum field healing is often used as a complimentary modality to Western medicine.

Ayurveda

Ayurveda medicine is one of the oldest forms of holistic medicine. Ayurveda originated in India over 3,000 years ago as of the writing of this text. The premise of Ayurveda is that wellness is a balance between body, mind, and spirit. Included in Ayurveda are the concepts of prana, nadis, and chakras. Prana is the universal life force that flows through every person. The Prana flows through the Nadis. Chakras process energy for the Nadis. The Ida, Pingala, and Sushumna are the major Nadis. They begin at the base of the spine with the Ida on the left side, the Pingala on the right side, and the Sushumna running up the middle. How easily this energy flows is based on balances or imbalances in the chakras.

Auras

Auras are the rainbow-colored energy field that surrounds us. The aura is invisible to the physical eye but can be perceived via claircognizance, psychometry, and clairvoyance. Aura energy is transmitted via the chakras. Each chakra empowers a layer of auric energy that responds to the color of the chakra. Disruptions in the auric field can be the cause of troublesome physical and emotional symptoms in individuals. People with clean auric fields and balanced chakras tend to report high levels of wellness.

Meridians

Meridians are rivers of subtle energy that flow through the human body. Discovered thousands of years ago, meridians are said to be the knowledge that led to Traditional Chinese Medicine. Concepts that relate to meridians are the five-phase theory, theories of yin and yang, the flow of emotions, internal and external sources of disease, and the cycle of life (Dale & Wehrman, 2017). The vital energy that flows through meridians pathways that are associated with specific organs in the body. Hand and foot massages are used by healers to tap into specific meridians to assist with physical body healing.

Chakras

The idea of chakras is part of a much larger philosophy of spiritual enlightenment. The concept is thousands of years old. Chakras were first described in Hindu knowledge, often used with other concepts like tantra and yoga. Although traditionally discussed as part of Hindu culture, chakras are referenced, using various names, by many cultures. The concept of chakras can be found in the Vedas, the Jewish Kabbalah, Incan traditions, as well as Taoism, Bonism, Sulfism, Buddhism, some tribal philosophies in North and South America, as well as with a few Christian sects.

Chakra energy does not revolve around the use of carbohydrates, adenosine triphosphate, or any other traditionally thought of food to function. Similar to physical body systems, chakras are always functioning but just like anything else, they may not be functioning *optimally*. An impaired chakra system can have a negative impact on the human body, mind, and spirit. Paying attention to this special energy system that resides in each one of us can help people live happier and more harmonious lives.

Kundalini

Kundalini is a feminine Sanskrit word that refers to the concept of life energy. Kundalini activates (awakens) the chakras and enables spiritual awakening and maturation. It is described as two serpents coiled at the base of the spinal cord lying dormant until awakened by specific practices directed at its awakening. Kundalini awakening can be a difficult process because as kundalini energy rises, unresolved issues and emotions come to the surface. This rising of kundalini energy into each chakra forces us to see the shadow self. Seeing the shadow self is important because truth requires seeing the entire self and not just the parts of self.

Shadow Self

Because you are reading this book, I assume that you are on some sort of journey. Perhaps it is a journey about learning yourself, learning about others, or a journey of curiosity about what besides the physical realm may exist. The shadow self is one of the things that exists beyond the physical realm. When thinking about the shadow self, think about what lies beneath the self that you project outward. The shadow self is where fears and desires that may be seen as abnormal to the masses resides. The shadow self is the part of a person that is not easily shared because it contains everything that may be considered taboo but must be acknowledged for the true self to be revealed.

Archetypes

Archetypes, first described by Carl Jung in the book *Archetypes of the Collective Unconscious* (1969), are patterns of human behavior. Archetypes represent the qualities in each one of us as a fixed pattern of human behavior. Various characters, such as a Fairy Godmother for example, have been used to represent archetypes throughout history. We respond to these characters in specific ways because they mirror parts of our own unconsciousness. Archetypes and chakras relate to one another because both represent and correlate with physical, emotional, psychological, and spiritual states of being (Wauters, 1997). In this text, a brief introduction to archetypes associated with each chakra will be discussed.

Meditation

For many centuries, beginning with ancient monks and mystics of India, people have *looked* within themselves in search of answers about life. Various methods have been used to connect with the human spirit. One of the most common methods is meditation. Meditation often involves focusing on a specific (statement) mantra, word, color, breath, or melody while allowing whatever else floats into consciousness to float away as easily as it entered your consciousness. A result of meditating was the realization that within each one of us exists an entire energy system that connects to the physical body but that is not the same as their physical body. Inside each one of us exists a way to work with the body at atomic level; without physically manipulating any part of the physical body. Meditation allows people to see themselves in the dominion of the psyche and to manage their physical body and psychological conditions (Lefebvre, 2017). Through constant meditation, these ancient monks and mystics discerned that, although there are many chakras, there are seven major energy systems in the human body. These seven major energy systems (chakras) are the ones discussed in this book.

Kundalini Yoga

Kundalini yoga was developed when practices that were heavy on ritual and included animal sacrifices fell out of favor with many people. Practitioners of Kundalini yoga believed that, because of confusion and materialism, enlightenment was and would continue to be difficult to attain during the cycle of human existence. Kundalini yoga methods were used to overcome this confusion and materialism by spiritualizing and creating light within the human physical body.

Kundalini is a life force energy that lies dormant at the base of the spine until awakened by various practices; kundalini yoga is one such practice. With kundalini yoga, the dormant energy is awakened and sent upward through the body toward the crown of the head then brought back down to the base of the spine. Along the way, this energetic loop of kundalini energy rises through energy centers in the body. These energy centers in the body are the *Chakras*. Once awakened, it is believed that chakras can have a positive impact on health and wellness in many areas of the human existence including physical, psychological, and spiritual realms.

Mindfulness

The word mindfulness refers to the act of being fully engaged in the moment. The concept of mindfulness is one where a person is conscious and aware of what is going on in their internal and external environments and is fully engaged with that environment. The busyness of everyday activities can decrease one's attention to being present and engaged in the moment; whereas, mindfulness activities and exercises can increase a person's desire and ability to be fully engaged in minute to minute activities. Mindfulness exercises can assist with raising a person's awareness about thoughts and emotions without judging them. Meditation and centering are commonly practice mindfulness exercises. Mindfulness exercises are commonly used for many issues, including pain relief and stress relief, either alone or as a compliment to western medicine.

CHAPTER 1

What Is a Chakra

Chakra, originally *cakra,* is Sanskrit word that means wheel (Joshi, 2016). Chakras are part of a philosophy about humanity's place in the spiritual hierarchy of the universe. They are the energy centers of our consciousness, functioning as valves that regulate energy as it flows through our energy system (Joshi, 2016). The way that we think and the way that we choose to respond to our environment reflect the state of our chakras and overall energy system (Joshi, 2016). Practitioners of complimentary therapies such as Reiki and Pranic Healing focus on chakras to assist clients with healing their mind and body. Research points to the use of complementary and alternative healing modalities as viable treatments for healing of the mind and body.

Theoretical Background: The Scientific Explanation

Chakras are vortexes that receive and process cosmic energy in a way that permit psychological, physical, and conscious functioning (Dale, 2016). Although commonly described as male or female chakras describing projection of energy (male) or receiving energy (female receptive), chakras receive scalar energy; energy that operates in a non-linear dimension of hyperspace (Joshi, 2016). The idea of chakra began in India as a part of the spiritual practice kundalini yoga. Chakras send information out from the person allowing the person to feel the intellectual state of cosmic consciousness; a state of enlightenment, elevation, or bliss (Joshi, 2016). Chakras are not physical in nature; instead they are part of consciousness that interact with the physical body through endocrine and nervous systems. Each of the seven major chakras is associated with one of the endocrine glands and a group of nerves; thus, the functioning of the chakras is linked to the gland or plexus associated with that chakra.

Energy exchange is an essential cornerstone of studies about human anatomy (Heymsfield, Bourgeois, & Thomas, 2017). Scientists have studied human energy exchange since civilization began. Studying about body heat production was and continues to be a common vehicle used to investigate human energy exchange. As early as the times of Hippocrates, Galen of Pergamon, and Sanctorius of Padua, man investigated to understand how energy works in the human body. People are energetic bodies that operate using physical energy that is created in part by subtle energy. According to the First Law of Thermodynamics, energy can be changed but it cannot be created or destroyed (Heymsfield, Bourgeois, & Thomas, 2017). Chakra energy works according to the First Law of Thermodynamics. Evidence of this is that although humans are primarily viewed for how they look, humans are a mass that is built of atoms containing electrons, protons, and neutrons. These protons, electrons, and neutrons make up the energy that produces the functions of the human body. Atoms are made of protons, electrons, and neutrons residing in electron shells. Variances in pressure impact the movement of atoms. For example, heat can speed up the movement of atoms and cold temperatures can slow down the movement of atoms. Atoms are the basic building block of everything including the cells that make up the organs and organ systems in the physical human body. Currently, we know that increases in body temperature increases the speed of some body functions and that decreasing body temperature slows down some physical processes. Vital sign measurement provides evidence of the impact of changes in temperature on the body and body systems.

Chakras are representative of your physical body and consciousness (Joshi, 2016). The seven main chakras discussed in this book can be divided into three categories: root, sacral, and solar plexus belong to the category of matter. Throat, third eye, and crown chakras belong to the category of spirit. The heart chakra sits in its own category because it is the chakra that bridges the gap between spirit and matter (Crowhurst, 2017). The heart chakra is where the ultimate love resides. With its active front and back sides, the heart chakra is the home of self-love that opens a person up to receive love from others and to give love to others.

The nervous system sends synaptic messages to work within the physical body to achieve the goal of physical homeostasis. The chakra system uses quantum tunneling to achieve its goal of sending messages to the energy system of the body. Quantum tunneling occurs when particles pass through an energy barrier that could not be accomplished in the classical physical environment governed by classical laws (Joshi, 2016). Quantum tunneling involves the quantum field and chakras much like the nervous system uses the brain, nerves, and spinal cord to accomplish its goal.

Complimentary healing methods assist clients when used alone and when used with medical treatment modalities to assist with symptom management and bringing a person into a state of physical, mental, psychological, and emotional homeostasis. For example, Pranic Healing, which uses the vital healing energy fields that surround the body and are within the body, has been shown to improve mild to moderate depression when used as a complimentary therapy (Rajagopal, Jois, Majgi, Kumar, & Shashidhar, 2018). Complimentary healing methods such as diaphragmatic breathing and progressive muscle relaxation reduce overall perceptions of stress and stress reactions in people experiencing various levels of stress. Diaphragmatic breathing and guided meditation are also used as a tool to alleviate pain in some individuals.

This section is substantially different than the rest of the book. As I write, the word *heavy* came to my conscious mind. But sometimes heavy is necessary to present a clear picture. A goal of this book is to present a clear picture. The science is all around us; literally, all we have to do is tap into it.

The term *chakra* refers to the spinning wheels of energy, a vortex of sorts, that reside in every person. As mentioned previously, chakras are not physical; instead, they are aspects of consciousness. Each chakra acts to connect the subtle bodies and transduce life force energy. Although not everyone can agree, there are an estimated 72,000 to 78,000 chakras in the human body. There are 7 major chakras, 21 minor chakras, 49 tiny chakras, and the rest are known as minute nano-chakras. Written records of mystic Indian philosophy, which include the kundalini concept, a concept that includes chakras in its teachings, appeared around 600 BC. About two hundred records of mystic Indian philosophy exist. The written records of mystic Indian philosophy are compiled in the Upanishads. The Upanishads are inspired utterances said to represent the height that the spirit of seers and saints of India experienced in contemplation of the Divine Spirit. The Upanishads are the last phase of the Vedic revelation, the truths revealed by God according to ancient seers of India, following the Mantras, Brahmanas, and the Aranyakas (Sarma, 1961). These written records continue to be an important part of mystic Indian philosophy.

The primary purpose of this book is to discuss the seven major chakras. The seven major chakras are positioned along the spine and interact with the physical body through the endocrine and nervous systems. The seven major chakras are the root chakra, sacral chakra, solar plexus chakra, heart chakra, throat chakra, third eye chakra, and the crown chakra.

Each chakra corresponds to a different part of who you are. Chakra energy moves from root to crown and each depends on the one before it for stability and harmony. Many people have unbalanced chakra systems but are not aware of the imbalances. Imbalanced in the chakra system manifest in spiritual, psychological, and physical systems.

Each chakra has its own color and vibration / vibratory tone. Each of the seven major chakras also has a geometric shape / platonic solid attached to them. Additionally, the first five elements are associated with an element. The color, vibration / vibratory tone, and geometric shape activate the chakra that it belongs to. Below is a table of this information for each of the major chakras. This information will be explored at length in the chapters of this book. The purpose of charts within this chapter are to provide an easy way to review basic chakra information.

Table 1. *The 7 Basic Chakras*

Chakra	Sanskrit Name	Location	Color	Geometric Shape	Vibratory Tone
Root	Muladhara	Base of the spine	Red	Hexahedron	Musical Note "C"
Sacral	Swadhisthana	Pelvis	Orange	Icosohedron	Musical Note "D"
Solar Plexus	Manipura	Epigastric Area of the Abdomen	Yellow	Tetrahedron	Musical Note "E"
Heart	Anahata	Center of Chest	Green	Octahedron	Musical Note "F"
Throat	Vishuddha	Throat	Blue	Dodecahedron	Musical Note "G"
Third Eye	Ajna	Forehead	Indigo	Merkaba	Musical Note "A"
Crown	Sahasrara	Top of the Head	Violet	Sphere	Musical Note "B"

As you become more exposed to the colors, shapes, emotions, and sensations associated with each chakra you will begin to notice their use in the environment and the reactions that each cause within yourself and others. As we explore each chakra you will be guided to pay attention to subtle signs within you that you will begin to recognize as meaning something to a specific situation or circumstance that you are or have been involved in . . . that flutter in your stomach when something was about to happen, your heart skipping a beat when that special person walks in the room, the calming effect of the color blue, and use of the words *seeing red* to describe anger are some examples of the phenomenon.

Imbalances

Just like every other body system, the desire of the chakra system is to be in balance. A healthy chakra system is one where every chakra is open to a healthy size, clear, and balanced. Imbalances in the chakra system can manifest in physical, emotional, and psychological symptoms. Chakras can become blocked or closed. They can also be *too* open. Individual imbalances impact the entire system. You will be provided with examples of these manifestations as we explore each individual chakra. For now, consider that chakra imbalances are the result of life experiences and our reactions to them. Blocked chakras are usually the result of a hurt of some kind. Closed chakras can be the result of blockage that have lasted too long or have had a major impact on the person. An example of a blockage leading to a closed chakra is broken heart leading to self-imposed isolation. Blown open chakras can be the result of overuse of the chakra. Blown means the chakra is stuck open; thus, it is very vulnerable to external influences. An example might be a baseball player who, over time, develops a rotator cuff tear or someone who uses their wrist and hand in a way that leads to carpel tunnel syndrome over time. In each of the preceding examples, repetitive use of the body part resulted in a weakness such that even normal use of the body part became problematic.

Power, Functions, and Tasks

As you will see throughout this book, each chakra has a different task. Each chakra is responsible for many things and has many tasks. The function of each chakra depends in some way on the chakra below it, with the exception of the root chakra because it is the first chakra and has an impact on the chakras above it. Additionally, as previously mentioned, the function of each chakra relates to the endocrine gland and nerve plexus with which the chakra is associated.

CHAPTER 2

The Root of the Matter

The root chakra is the foundation of the seven-chakra system; the foundation for physical and spiritual energy. The root chakra resides at the base of the spine and puts forth its energy through the lower part of the body including the hips, legs, and feet. This chakra aids in grounding—the feeling that we are all connected and that we are a part of our environments. The color associated with the root chakra is red. The root chakra is associated with the basic survival needs safety and security. Work ethic and ability are also associated with this chakra. The root chakra controls the energy for kinesthetic feeling and movement; as such, the desire to move is associated with the root chakra. The root chakra aligns with material success, knowledge, self-assurance, and constancy. Archetypes that relate to the root chakra are the mother and the victim. Emotional issues for this chakra, should they arise, revolve around grounding.

Balanced

A person with a healthy root chakra exhibits behaviors that show they are grounded and fearless. They tend to focus on their *chosen* tasks and spend little time being concerned about the impact that material things and people have on them as individuals. Despite this freeness, they are not compulsive and careless; instead they operate from a place of empowerment. People with healthy root chakras are easily able to empower others because they enjoy empowering others they are literally filled with happiness and success.

Imbalanced

A person with a closed, blocked, or weak root chakra exhibits low levels of activity and enthusiasm which they attribute to lethargy. Oftentimes they complain of depression [as evidenced by finding little pleasure in physical activities and things they once found pleasurable] and may have physical symptoms including low back pain, leg pain, and problems with their immune systems. These are people who require constant stimulation from a person or other source outside of themselves. Feelings of flightiness, being disconnected from reality, and doubt are often seen in a person with an unbalanced root chakra. A person with an unbalanced root chakra finds it difficult to be loyal to themselves and others. They often have very unstable relationships as a result.

Sometimes people with imbalanced root chakras complain of being angry all the time. To others, a person with an imbalanced root chakra may also appear to be angry all the time and the anger may not have an apparent cause. Sometimes people with imbalanced root chakras may be branded with mental illnesses, including personality disorders. Although a mental illness can be a cause for angry and aggressive behaviors, people with blown open root chakras can also exhibit these behaviors and as such investigation is warranted. Investigating for root chakra imbalances is important in people who exhibit aggressive, stifling, and oppressive behaviors when interacting with others.

CHAPTER 3

Yippee Hippee

The Sacral Chakra is located below the naval and above the pubic bone; around the hip area. The color associated with the sacral chakra is orange. It is known as the water chakra. The sacral chakra controls the flow of energy through the body. It operates as the gravity center and the center of the life force of the body. This chakra is female receptive; receiving energy from the root chakra. Charisma and magnetism reside in the sacral chakra. These characteristics can be positive or negative depending on the state a person's state of being.

Our ability to reproduce, sexual love-pleasure-and desire, as well as energy about emotions and relationships reside in the sacral chakra. Emotional and relationship energy living in the sacral chakra include giving, receiving, and harmony. Creativity also resides here and is often seen as change, movement, and the integration of new ideas. A goal of working with this chakra is to adopt an attitude of surrender; surrendering to the thought that we are part of all that is around us. Archetypes related to the sacral chakra are the emperor / empress or the martyr. Classically, the emperor / empress represent the mother and father of creativity. Emotional concerns that relate to the sacral chakra are about assuredness and well-being.

Balanced

A person with a balanced sacral chakra is a joy to be around because they enjoy life. They embrace creativity and their sexuality. People with balanced root chakras handle change easily because they are flexible in body and mind. This flexibility allows them to stay grounded instead of becoming fixated on controlling things they have no control over.

Imbalanced

A person with a closed, blocked, or weak sacral chakra often appears confused, frustrated, and / or bitter. Their behaviors are easily influenced by others because they excessively depend on others. A person with a blocked sacral chakra may be absent in personal relationships or may not have significant relationships with others because they tend to fear sensuality and / or sexuality.

CHAPTER 4

The Nerves Have It

The solar plexus chakra is located between the rib cage and navel (stomach area). The color associated with the solar plexus chakra is yellow. This chakra is the first of the relationship chakras. It is the core or *center of who you* are; as such, value systems, criticisms, and support reside here. It is known as the fire chakra. In addition to being the first of the relationship chakras, it is the energy distribution center of the chakra system. The solar plexus works like a power station. Tapping into the power of the solar plexus during the day can diminish episodic moments of fatigue.

Physically, the solar plexus chakra corresponds to pancreas and controls immune and digestive systems. As previously mentioned, the solar plexus is positioned in the stomach area. The stomach is the second brain because second to the brain, the stomach has the highest concentration of nerves in the human body. Psychologically, the solar plexus is the seat of confidence. It is also where your ego resides. Spiritually, the solar plexus is the seat of soul. The solar plexus is a masculine chakra that projects will, strength, force, and determination, out into the world and then back to you.

Archetypes related to the solar plexus chakra are the warrior or the servant. Emotional issues that can arise related to the solar plexus involve power and self-worth.

Balance

A person with a balanced solar plexus is strong. Physically, they tend to be able to fight infections and have few, if any, allergic reactions. They are also able to use the nutrients they ingest more efficiently. They are able to live without fear of violating rules, dictums, and dogmas that belong to others. People with balanced solar plexus chakras often discuss feelings of *freeness* as they become more comfortable with interpreting the world around them through their own thoughts and emotions. The spirit of knowing who one is and embodying this spirit encourages integrity and unchanging principles that dictate words, actions, and deeds.

For a person with a balanced solar plexus keeping commitments to self and others is important. The more they keep their commitments the stronger their attitude of achievement becomes until ultimately achievement is replaced with success; happiness. What was once seen as obstacles become opportunities to be successful. When your solar plexus chakra is in balance it is easy to project authority, self-control, and awakening into the world. A balanced solar plexus makes transformation desirable and easy. People with balanced solar plexus chakras stand out as leaders for many reasons including their humor, radiance, laughter, and warmth.

Imbalance

The solar plexus chakra can become imbalanced. Symptoms of a closed, blocked, or weak solar plexus chakra can be physical, spiritual, or emotional in nature. In fact, a person can have symptoms that includes more than one of the aforementioned natures at the same time. Common physical complaints include low infection tolerance, hormone issues, and food intolerances. Spiritually, a person with an imbalanced solar plexus chakra tends to give up easily because they lack the strength required to do what they are supposed to do. People with a solar plexus chakra imbalance function from a place of fear; fear of the impact their ideas, decisions, and behaviors may have on the lives of others. Even though a person with an imbalanced solar plexus chakra may sacrifice themselves for the needs of others, they fear living their life in a way that the pleasure of others is placed before their own needs. Just like the root and sacral chakras, the solar plexus can become stuck open. A person with a stuck open (aka blown open) solar plexus chakra appears either as out of control or exhibits actions commonly associated with an inflated ego.

CHAPTER 5

The Heart of the Matter

The heart chakra is located in the chest area near the center of the breastbone. The heart chakra is associated with the *thymus* gland. In humans, the thymus gland is usually atrophying and is replaced by fatty tissue in late adolescence (Nayak, Kumar, Aithal, Shetty, Sirasangandla, & Guru, 2015). The heart chakra is the central chakra. It is the bridge between physical and spiritual lives. The heart chakra is a feminine receptive chakra that receives and feels all that is in the internal and external environments. The heart chakra is often the area of greatest wounding because it balances our inner self with the external environment by regulating our interactions with the world around us. *Colors* associated with the heart chakra are green and pink. It is the relationships people have with themselves, others, and the source of everything. Divine unconditional love, empathy, and oneness with everything originate in the heart chakra because it is the headquarters of acceptance, openness, balance, and contentment. Remember when I said, "the heart chakra is associated with the thymus gland" and "the thymus gland usually atrophies and is replaced with fatty tissue in late adolescence"? What if this is because we become more closed with our experiences?

As mentioned above, the heart chakra has two colors associated with it. There are two colors because the heart chakra has two parts; kind of like a front and back. The front is the giving side. This side is where we give love to everything in the environment including people. The color associated with the front side is green. The back side is the receiving side. This is where the love we give ourselves sits. The color associated with the back side is pink. Although both sides are important, the backside is the gateway to being able to efficiently use the front side because self-love, receiving love from and of self has to come first. Being good at giving love requires we are also comfortable with giving ourselves love. Archetypes related this chakra are the lover or the actor. Are you loving or acting like you are loving? Emotional issues related to the heart chakra relate to the ability to give or receive love.

Balanced

People with balanced heart chakras seem relaxed and accepting of others and of life in general. They have easy interactions with others and are at ease to meet the demands of the world without overlooking their own needs because they easily realize when their needs are being compromised. They easily interact with others and easily meet the demands of the world without compromising their own needs because they have awareness of when their needs are being compromised. Finding balance between their inner and outer needs is easy for people with balanced heart chakras because they are open. Their openness is even evident in their posture. Although the degree of openness does not necessarily correlate with how erect the posture is, they stand erect with their shoulders back and their chests out because they are open to love and loving. People with balanced heart chakras can see the Creator of everything in everyone because they see everyone through the eyes of love which allows them to see that everything and everyone is connected. The ability to see the connection is why people with balanced heart chakras tend to have deep bonds with others.

Imbalanced

An imbalanced heart chakra is the result of holding on to emotions of sadness, regret, and unhappiness that do not serve us. Just like a balanced heart chakra can be seen in the posture of the person, posture is an indicator of an imbalanced heart chakra. People with imbalanced heart chakras tend to have a tense upper torso and often sit with their arms folded so nothing can get in or out. They tend to have poor or weak relationships and receive no enjoyment from being touched by others or from touching others. Oftentimes, they resist handshakes and hugs and give loose ones if they do give a handshake or hug. All relationships are an issue for people with imbalanced heart chakras, but intimate ones are the most difficult. In relationships, people with heart chakra imbalances tend to function as controlling or being controlled. They also tend to find difficultly to accept things, including compliments, gifts, and affections, from others.

This concludes our discussion about the lower chakras. Although the heart chakra is technically not a lower chakra, because it is the central or middle, the heart chakra was included in this section because it is not the same as the upper or subtle vibration chakras.

In the next three chapters, the subtle vibration chakras will be discussed. The subtle vibration chakras require greater level of listening and sensitivity. Unlike the physical world where definitive indicators of needs and changes exist, the subtle vibration chakras are connected to an invisible subtle realm that speaks to each of us in dreams, ideas, whispers, and energies.

CHAPTER 6

Thinking It and Saying It

The name of the throat chakra describes its location; at the throat. The color associated with the throat chakra is blue. It is known as the ether chakra. Ether is the element that binds the elements of earth, air, water, and fire together with physical and spiritual worlds. The throat chakra is the home of expression. The throat chakra functions as the voice of the body; allowing energy from the other chakras to be expressed. The throat chakra is a masculine chakra that allows projection of spiritual energy and ideas into the world, corresponding with the thyroid gland. The thyroid gland regulates metabolism.

The throat chakra deals with unconditional truth. As such, it is important in sharing your authentic self. Sharing your authentic self can be challenging because of requiring openness and the projection of truth regardless without considering how others may perceive. The positioning of the throat chakra, just above your heart chakra, is important because of a direct connection between the throat and heart chakras. The term *speaking from the heart* illustrates this connection. When people speak from their hearts, they are able to connect with people and move them to action. People known for their creativity and speaking ability possess strong heart chakras.

Words are spells in that words impact people. Always remember to choose your words wisely. Also consider how you use words when speaking to yourself and others. Speak your truth consciously. Through the words we speak we impact the way others think, behave, and feel. Using words, such as affirmations and mantras, a person creates reality because affirmations and mantras bring in the *vibrations* that align with how the person wants to feel. Something as simple as replacing the word *if* with the word *when* changes the vibration of what comes next in the sentence or thought and speaks loudly to your subconscious; thus, allowing the ability to create the reality you want to see.

Because we speak to ourselves constantly, through inner dialogue, we have the ability to live in our own worlds of truth or delusions. Being honest with ourselves during our inner dialogue sessions encourages a life of true happiness because of opening doors for us to see that we have much to share with the world around us. A challenging aspect of strengthening the throat chakra is our desire for instant gratification or substantiation. Neither instant gratification nor instant substantiation may happen. As previously mentioned, the throat chakra is one of the subtle body chakras, so one has to pay close attention as the vibrations begin to rise.

Balance

People with balanced throat chakras easily express their thoughts and emotions. They easily share their personal truth by communicating their ideas and beliefs to themselves and others. They appear unburdened to others because energy freely flows within them at physical and spiritual levels. The free-flowing energy of a balanced throat chakra is the result from the energy from the preceding chakras flowing freely up into the throat chakra. People with balanced throat chakras are true communicators; because they speak with kindness, knowledge, and wisdom other people them. People with balanced throat chakras are confident in their abilities because they are honest and genuine with themselves and others. A profound sense of inner peace belongs to people with balanced throat chakras because they are comfortable with sharing their authentic self with others. Simple debates rarely turn into arguments for people with balanced throat chakras because people with balanced throat chakras are comfortable enough to debate without attaching emotion. Archetypes related to the throat chakra are the communicator or the silent child. Emotional issues that relate to the throat chakra center around effective communication.

Imbalance

People with imbalanced throat chakras have many physical and emotional expressions of the imbalanced chakra. Physically, they complain of sore throats, stiff necks, and headaches. To others, People with imbalanced throat chakras appear stiff because they have clinched jaws or pinched lips. Stammering, stuttering, and loss of words can be a problem for people with imbalanced throat chakras because they habitually lie to themselves and others out of fear and distrust about the intentions of others. Verbalizations of feeling isolated and misunderstood are also common for people with imbalanced throat chakras. They may also project symptoms of imbalanced foot, sacral, solar plexus, or heart chakras because blockage of this chakra blocks the energy flow from the other centers below it. The symptoms are the result of them not expressing their authentic feelings and truth. A person with a closed throat chakra is not expressive and a person with a blown open throat chakra tends to babble and finds it difficult to be quiet.

CHAPTER 7

Seeing IS Believing

The third eye chakra, also known as the brow chakra, is located in the center of the forehead. The color associated with the third eye chakra is indigo. The third eye chakra is associated the pituitary gland. The pituitary gland is a control center for the physical body in control of hormonal regulation. Just like the solar plexus, the third eye chakra is a relationship chakra. The relationship that works through the third eye is the one we have with ourselves. The third eye chakra is a command center for understanding. This chakra allows the ability to see the meaning of information collected through our five senses.

The third eye chakra is a feminine receptive chakra whose domains is the mind and learning. The third eye chakra directs sight and awareness of ourselves and the world around us. It is through this chakra that the ability to critically think resides. Scientists, researchers, and scholars have strong third eye chakras. Everyone who is inquisitive uses their third eye chakra to discern truth from fiction. The third eye chakra becomes closed when people close themselves off gaining new information; whereas, seeking information opens it.

The third eye chakra works hand-in-hand with the throat chakra because you must seek the truth before you can speak the truth. Learning is the domain or the third eye. The third eye is the seat of higher perception and knowing; as such it is the place where intuition resides. Intuition brings information based on the power of the mind combined with a spiritual connection to the world of ideas and ethers. The third eye is where you make decisions and build your beliefs.

The third eye chakra is where a person creates their reality by manifesting the results of internal dialogue. It the source of belief systems because the third eye is where we develop how we see the world. The third eye chakra is where we can adjust what we see to what we want to see in the world. If a person does not like the world they see, they can rewrite the images they see by internalizing and projecting love and confidence because with the creation of new internal beliefs your outer world will follow.

Maintaining positive thoughts are important for this chakra because of the ease of getting caught up in the lower vibrational thoughts that can cloud a person's mind. Like the physical body, the mind is a personal space and we have to be careful what we let in. When we fill the body with poor nutrition, physical illness can occur. When we fill the mind with poor low vibrational thought, illnesses in the mind can occur.

Meditation is important for the third eye chakra because it creates stillness within; allowing a person to discern fact from fiction. When meditating for the third eye chakra, contemplate what you see because meditation and contemplation will assist with the development of intuitive knowledge. People who master the third eye chakra are able to find meaning in dreams, symbols, and various energies in internal and external environments. Learning to perceive things through the third eye chakra allows you to notice things about yourself and the world that you have not noticed before. The insight that is provided by mastery of the third eye chakra leads to peace of mind and soul fulfillment. Archetypes related to the third eye chakra are the intuitive or the intellectual. Emotional issues that relate to this chakra are about the use of information for health and / or happiness (Wauters, 1997). Thinking is believing and this is the chakra where thoughts and perceptions matter most.

Balanced

A person with a balanced third eye chakra sees things clearly and understands what they see. They interpret visual cues easily because they have a high level of discernment. They are open to learning because their thoughts and internal dialogue are healthy and strong. To others, a person with a balanced third eye chakra appears observant and quiet. Having a balanced third eye chakra allows a person to control the energy flow in all the chakras.

Imbalanced

Imbalances in the third chakra impact the whole person. Third eye chakra imbalances cause difficulty with command of body and thought. A person with an imbalanced third eye chakra has trouble making sense of the things they encounter. They appear confused because they have difficulty with knowing what is important. Physical complaints include earaches, headaches, and vision problems. They resist new ideas and information. Because they lose access to their intuition, they have trouble with working through problems.

The most significant third eye chakra imbalance is a blown open chakra. A person with a blown open third eye chakra appears out of control. They are constantly looking for new ideas and information simply for the sake of finding new ideas and information. They constantly think about any and everything but make no practical use of their thoughts or any information obtained from their research.

CHAPTER 8

Crowning Yourself

The crown chakra is the gateway to the universe and the universal law that expands beyond our physical bodies. It is located at the top of the head and points upward. The color associated with the crown chakra is purple. Purple is the color of royalty and is the highest color of light that the human eye can see. The color purple links to the realm of spirituality that is hidden from the human eye. The purple of the crown relates to surrendering and learning how to let go. About how to let go of ego and trust in a higher intelligence that wants to guide you. The crown chakra receives and downloads information from the source of all things. It controls our thinking and our response to the world around us. The crown chakra is the source of spirituality, beliefs, and values.

The crown chakra corresponds to the pineal gland. The pineal gland is in the center of your head. It looks like a pine cone. It secretes DMT (dream hormone) and melatonin. At death, near death, drug trips, DMT floods the brain and produces a vision to the person. The pineal gland can transmit and receive the waves of different realms. Meditation is very important to the pineal gland.

The crown chakra connects us to a higher plane of existence by extending our energy beyond the boundaries of our bodies. Allowing for awareness beyond space and time, the crown chakra connects us to infinite oneness and everything that ever was and everything that ever will be. Herein lies the source of higher information and universal truth, as well as the source of physical coordination and our relationship with movement through life.

Mastering of the crown chakra can only happen after the chakras below it have been mastered. The crown chakra represents openness and willingness to be part of a greater plan than the one associated with the human ego. The crown chakra unifies higher self and human personality because it is a continuity of consciousness. Divine wisdom, idealism, inspiration, and spiritual will reside in the crown chakra. The crown chakra is where strong leaders gather the guidance and wisdom that helps lead others.

The crown chakra balances out the solar plexus chakra because it provides the spiritual strength and will to drive a person forward. Similar to the third eye chakra, meditation is important to the crown chakra. It is with meditation that a person can surrender. The surrender associated with a balanced crown chakra allows for efficiency in actions because answers to issues come when we are still and can hear the higher vibrations that resonate with true peace. Meditating and surrendering calms an overactive mind; however, surrender and acceptance can feel foreign or difficult because of the ease to feel lost when a person is not in control of situations that impact them. Throughout life experiences, parents, and teachers teach the importance of being in control of one's life and to work hard to find the answers and gain control when a person feels out of control.

Using the crown chakra effectively happens when a person asks for something and gives thanks for receiving it even when they have not received it yet. Giving thanks is possible for a person with a balanced crown chakra because they know that if they are asking for something honestly and for the greatest good it will manifest into reality. They know that after asking and thanking, the person waits and listens for the words they are supposed to hear. The answer may come during a meditation or from a place or person close to the person who has made the request. The answer may also come from a random person, place, or sign of some sort.

Some people use substances to reach the enlightenment associated with mastering the crown chakra. Although using various substances may work because some substances relax inhibitions, the effect wears off when the substance is no longer in use. Meditation and spiritual development are what gives a person the ability to access this area at any time. Developing a spiritual practice or ritual connects a person to the infinite universe; a universe of endless possibilities.

Signs and symbols are a way that spirit connects us to each other and to the universe. Common signs and symbols include random numbers, colors, birds, butterflies, and dragonflies. Historically, learning to interpret signs and symbols was an important skill in many cultures. In some cultures, interpreting signs continues to be important today. Sign and symbol interpretation are the intuition's way of speaking. Nonlogical sources, such as sign and symbol interpretation, provide information that allows for discernment of what needs to happen next; however, it should not be used to replace logic. Instead, interpretation can and should be used as a tool to direct a person on the soul's true path. Archetypes associated with the crown chakra are the guru and the egotist. Emotional issues that arise related to the crown chakra are about the highest spiritual awareness (Wauters, 1997). Connecting with the universe allows a person to live in a world where they realize that endless possibilities exist.

Balanced

When the crown chakra is balanced and open, a person is connected to the world. They realize what seems like coincidences are not coincidences because there is no such thing. They have feelings of being balanced and know where and how they relate to the universe. Adapting to change is easy for a person with a balanced crown chakra because they understand life and see people, situations, and circumstances as they truly are. A person with a balanced crown chakra easily handles issues because they know that issues and concerns are just a part of life. They live in the present and are mindful because they do not have any desire to hang on to the past. A person with a balanced crown chakra listens to the inner voice for guidance and obeys the inner voice for the greatest good of all because they are open to receiving information from the universe.

Imbalanced

A person with an imbalanced crown chakra may appear clumsy and uncoordinated. They may stumble in physical movement and thought; tending to appear uninspired and displaying rigid thought patterns or appearing spiritually lost. This is because a person with an imbalanced crown chakra is unsure of who they are and why they exist. They have difficulty with ideas, goals, and relationships because they do not understand them.

Significant issues for this chakra occur when the chakra is either closed or blown open. When the crown chakra is closed a person is cut off from spirit. They complain about how awful life is for them compared to the life of others. They are not open to receiving guidance, do not trust the universe or a higher power, and feel as if the universe has abandoned them. People with blown open crown chakras continuously look for answers. They develop rituals and use them all day every day. The overuse of rituals leads to them receiving so much energy and information from the universe, without the ability to interpret, that the information they receive from the universe is not useful to them.

CHAPTER 9

Stability

As discussed in previous chapters, chakras can become imbalanced. Although healing practitioners can assist with chakra balancing, the process requires work on the part of the individual to maintain the balance. It is also possible for a person to balance his or her own chakra. Treatment modalities such as Reiki and crystal healing balance chakras and maintain them in a balanced state. Individuals can use meditative techniques, affirmations, and mantras to create balance, rebalance, and to maintain balance in the chakras. In this chapter, we will review some common manifestations of imbalances and some exercises to assist with imbalances in each of the seven chakras previously discussed.

Throughout this text, meditation has been mentioned as a tool to bring and maintain stability in the body and mind by allowing a person's higher self to emerge. Through the use of meditation, a person is able to attune the mind and body to a spiritual source. Meditation is a devotional exercise that is works to calm the body and mind. Meditation helps with focus, concentration, cleansing, and clarity in individuals and groups of individuals. The focus, concentration, cleansing, and clarity provided by meditation allows a person to learn his or herself, be comfortable with his or herself, and express his or her true self with ease because with meditation a person develops a greater sense of trust in his or her intuition. Meditation is generally divided into two types. The focus of one type is to reach a state where the practitioner feels as if they are dissolving into nothingness. The goal of the second type is to reach a feeling of oneness with the universe, source, or creator of all things. For stabilizing, balancing, and maintaining balanced chakras, meditation is done by making the imbalanced chakra the focus of attention during meditation. Meditating with chakras can be done either by beginning with the lowest chakra, the root chakra, and moving up until the highest chakra, the crown chakra, is reached or by meditating on a specific chakra that is out of balance.

As discussed previously:

- Protons, electrons, and neutrons reside in electron shells.
- Protons, electrons, and neutrons, combined together make atoms; thus, atoms are energetic bodies.
- Atoms are the basic building block of everything, including the cells in the human body.
- The cells in the human body contain energy.
- Human beings are energetic bodies that operate using physical and subtle energy systems.

Root

People with root chakra issues are always looking for conflict in their environment. Because the root chakra is the first chakra, working on the root chakra involves working on the chakra and the chakras above it. Exercises to create and maintain balance in the root chakra focus on working to see your true self and what helps you feel safe and grounded. When an imbalance is noted, realizing what you need and how to meet the need is paramount. Meditation, surrounding yourself with people who have balanced root chakras, and taking care of your internal and external environment can assist with balancing the root chakra and maintaining its balance. Meditation using crystals that are red, like red jasper, can assist with root chakra maintenance. Affirmations including: (a) I am safe, (b) I am secure, and (c) I love my body are helpful when working with the root chakra. Mantras for the root chakra are Mul Mantra to eliminate fear and Lam. Also, remember to take care of your physical body. Taking time to eat right, pamper yourself, and exercise regularly help develop and maintain a healthy root chakra. Remember we are often known by the company we keep so surrounding yourself with people who have balanced root chakras allows the ability to share root chakra energy.

Sacral

People with sacral chakra issues are inflexible and have a difficult time adapting to their environment. Problems with pelvic organs, like urinary tract infections and ovarian cysts can be related to sacral chakra imbalances. Lower back pain are also common complaints for people with sacral chakra imbalances. Problems with creativity and the ability to expression emotions are often the result of an imbalanced sacral chakra. Exercises to create and maintain balance in the sacral chakra involves working with the root chakra as well as the solar plexus chakra. Meditation using crystals that are orange, like carnelian, can assist with sacral chakra maintenance. Affirmations including: (a) I am creative, (b) I am worthy of love, and (c) I am worthy of a healthy life are helpful when working with the sacral chakra. Mantras for the sacral chakra are Adi Shakti to call upon the divine force of creativity and to balance and heal the chakra and vam, the seed mantra that activates the chakra.

Solar Plexus

People with solar plexus chakra issues are anxious and are afraid of making decisions. Digestive and metabolic concerns are common for people with solar plexus imbalances. They may also use food as a comfort measure to assist with feelings of inadequacy and low self-worth. Exercises to create and maintain balance in the solar plexus chakra include working with this chakra and with the sacral and heart chakras. Meditation using crystals that are yellow, like tiger eye and citrine, can assist with solar plexus maintenance. Affirmations including: (a) I can do all things, (b) I am empowered, and (c) I lovingly accept and appreciate myself are helpful when working with the solar plexus chakra. Mantras for the solar plexus chakra are Har, which calls on the source of the universe and everything in it and activates the solar plexus, and ram, the seed mantra that also activates the chakra.

Heart

People with heart chakra issues are unloving of themselves and others. Heart, lung, and blood pressure issues are common for people with heart chakra imbalances. They may also appear cynical and manipulative. Exercises to create and maintain balance in the heart chakra include working with this chakra as well as the solar plexus and throat chakras. Forgiveness of oneself and others and realizing that learning is a part of life are essential to balancing the heart chakra. Meditating with green crystals, like aventurine and jade, as well as pink crystals, like rose quartz, can assist with heart chakra maintenance. Affirmations including: (a) I love, (b) I am loved, and (c) I am proud of who I am are helpful when working with the heart chakra. Mantras for the heart chakra are Guru Ram Das, to call in loving protection and open and heal the heart, and yam, the seed mantra that activates the chakra.

Throat

People with throat chakra issues hide behind falsehood. They have problems telling the truth and expressing their truth. Neck, throat, and thyroid problems are common for people with throat chakra imbalances. They may also have a difficult time accepting new ideas and listening to others express their truth. Exercises to create and maintain balance in the throat chakra include working with this chakra and the heart chakra, journaling at least 20 minutes per day using pen and paper, reflective writing, and meditation. Journaling and reflective writing encourage honesty with self. Meditating with blue crystals, like blue lace agate and lapis lazuli, can assist with throat chakra maintenance. Affirmations including: (a) I speak truth, (b) I communicate my truth easily, and (c) I express myself lovingly are helpful when working with the throat chakra. Mantras for the heart chakra are Humee Hum, to open and soothe the chakra, and ham, the seed mantra that activates the chakra.

Third Eye

People with third eye issues can be either egocentric or uncertain. The difference depends on whether the chakra is blown open or closed respectively. Vision problems, hearing problems, and headaches are also common complaints for people with third eye imbalances. Exercises to create and maintain balance involve working with this chakra and the third eye chakra. Meditating with violet or indigo crystals, like sodalite and amethyst, can assist with third eye chakra maintenance. Affirmations including: (a) I am aware, (b) I open myself to my inner guidance, and (c) I create clarity and unlimited vision for myself. Mantras for the third eye chakra are Ong Sohung, to connect come into a state of expanded knowingness and OM, the seed mantra that activates the energy of the chakra.

Crown Chakra

People with crown chakra issues are metaphorically lost; having no sense of purpose. Neurological disorders are common for people with crown chakra imbalances. This highest chakra of the physical body so while meditation with crystals like clear quartz and amethyst are very beneficial and a great place to start, advanced meditation techniques like guided meditation, visualization, and transcendental meditation will accelerate the functioning of this chakra. Prayer is way to strengthen the crown chakra. Sincerity and intention determine how / when your prayers are answered and the effectiveness of your prayers. Practice observing the things around you. Affirmations including: (a) I am, (b) I am love, and (c) I am worthy are helpful for working with the crown chakra. Mantras for the crown chakra are Waheguru, to connect to infinite experiences and OM, the seed chakra that activates the energy of the chakra. Affirmations, mantras, crystals, and essential fragrances that can be used as part of a meditative practice when working with the chakras is listed in Table 2. The fragrances are often used to set the mood in a room where meditative practices occur.

Table 2. ***Chakra Healing Aids***

Chakra	Affirmation	Mantra	Crystal	Essential Oil/ Fragrance
Crown	I am I am love I am worthy	Wahegure OM Shrim (Shreem)	Amethyst Clear Quartz Ametrine	Frankincense Lime Rose
Third Eye	I am aware I open myself to my inner guidance I create clarity and unlimited vision for myself	Ong Sohung OM Shrim (Shreem)	Amethyst Cinnabar Fluorite	Lavender Jasmin Sandalwood
Throat	I speak truth I communicate my truth easily I express myself lovingly	Humee Hum Brahm Hum Ham	Blue Lace Agate Lapis Lazuli Moonstone	Eucalyptus Chamomile Frankincense
Heart	I am loved I love I am proud of who I am	Guru Ram Das Yam Hrim (Hreem)	Rose Quartz Green Aventurine	Rose Neroli Jasmin
Solar Plexus	I can do all things I am empowered I lovingly accept and appreciate myself	Har Ram Krim (Kreem)	Yellow Tiger Eye Citrine	Blood Orange Cinnamon Peppermint
Sacral	I am creative I am worthy of love I am worthy of a healthy life	Adi Shakti Vam Krim (Kreem)	Amber Carnelian Sunstone	Neroli Sandalwood Patchouli
Root	I am safe I am secure I love my body	Mul Mantra Lam Krim (Kreem)	Hematite Red Jasper Bloodstone	Patchouli Myrrh Cedarwood

CHAPTER 10

Paired Chakras and Beyond

Previously, discussions included the basic 7 chakras, what can happen with them, and ways to balance and maintain balance of them. The focus of this chapter is to provide information that expands on the previous chapters and encourages further learning about chakras and how they work to maintain health and wellness.

Paired Chakras

Paired chakras, called *paired chakra channels*, are chakras the work together to produce an outcome that is either stronger than the outcome of either single chakra in the pair or an outcome that is different than the outcome of either single chakra in the pair. Paired chakra channels are the root / heart channel, the sacral / throat channel, the solar plexus / crown channel, the green / pink channel, the root / crown, the sacral / third eye, and the solar plexus / throat channel.

The root/heart chakra, also called *the green / red channel,* controls feelings of safety and security. A balanced heart chakra acts as a guardian shield; guarding against dark energy. When the heart chakra is balanced and open to giving self love, love to others, and open to receiving love from others, the root chakra feels safe. When the heart chakra is unbalanced, and a person does not have the ability to give or receive love, the root chakra engages to protect the person. Working together, the root and heart chakras create a sense of loving, belonging, safety, and security for the person.

The sacral / throat chakra channel, also called the *orange / blue* channel, controls feelings and expression of feelings. In this context, feelings and the expression of feelings are not the same because a person can be capable of feeling something that they are unable to express or that they are uncomfortable with expressing to others. Women often have stronger sacral / throat chakra channels because they tend to receive more encouragement, from others, to express their feelings and vulnerabilities than men are encouraged to express their feelings and vulnerabilities.

The solar plexus / crown chakra channel, also called the *yellow / purple* chakra channel, relates to faith. The throat and crown chakras balance each other when they work together. The crown chakra receives messages from a higher power and is able to act on the solar plexus in a way that is calming. A balanced solar plexus / crown chakra provides a sense of peace, even when situations and circumstances are less than peaceful.

The *green / pink* chakra channel is different than the chakra channels previously discussed in this chapter because unlike the other chakra channels, the green / pink chakra channel involves only one chakra. The green / pink chakra is both sides of the heart. The green side of the channel directs love to yourself and the pink side of the channel directs love to and receives love from others.

In addition to the chakra channels, the chakra system has some chakras that work together in some way to form a connection that exerts influence on the energy body system. Channels include the root to crown chakra connection, the sacral to third eye connection, and the solar plexus to throat connection. The focus of the connection is truth. The solar plexus to throat connection is the pathway provides a connection between physical and spiritual truths. The sacral to third eye connection focusses on reality. The third eye provides the vision that manifests reality. Together they allow a person to see the truth and create the reality as a manifestation in their life. The solar plexus to throat connection focuses on the connection between expression and power. The solar plexus to throat connection work together to balance emotions and encourage the expression of emotions in a healthy way because in a healthy state the connection is empowering. The solar plexus to throat connection allows a person to express their true self in a way that they and others see the power they have and are able to project into the world.

Ethnicity

Conversations about ethnicity, belonging to a specific group based on common culture, are usually reserved for hard sciences, sociology, and historical discussion. Rarely is ethnicity brought up in conversations about subtle energies; however, ethnicity does have a role in discussions about chakras and subtle energy. Throughout history entire societies have chosen to strengthen different chakras. Focusing on the specific chakras, whether on purpose or by accident provided a means of survival. This section includes exploration of the effects of strong chakras on specific ethnicities.

The Root Chakra

People of African descent commonly present as the most grounded and athletic. Of all ethnicities, people of African descent tend to prevail in tasks requiring strength and speed because they are naturally stronger than other races. Throughout thousands of years, this strength has been used for survival. The result of the drive for survival, in this ethnic group, is a strong root chakra.

The Throat Chakra

Throughout history, continuous conflict and scarce resources on European continents led to an emphasis on prioritizing conflict. Because of continuous warring and constant competition, people of European descent became will power oriented and strengthening of the ego occurred.

The end result is that people of European descent have strong throat chakras.

The Heart Chakra

The Native American descent name applies to a large group of people originating in the Americas. Their traditions are steeped in practices that place emphasis on connective oneness between man and earth. People of Native American descent are very grounded and open hearted. As a result of the man earth connection in people of Native American descent, they have very strong heart chakras.

The Asian culture is one of majestic examination. The Asian culture places value on intelligence. For members of this cultural group, intelligence includes gaining knowledge and being able to use the knowledge obtained in ways that strengthen the collective. There is a great emphasis on collectivism for this cultural group because survival meant they had to work together to produce what was needed. As a result of having to work together to maintain the collective more cohesiveness was maintained. The thought that everything done is for the good of the group is why people of Asian descent tend to have strong heart chakras.

Third Eye and Crown Chakras

The Hindu Indian culture places emphasis on the spirit of man. People of Hindu Indian ethnicity value their spiritual leaders as sources who connect with the divine and use this connection to provide leadership. As a result of the emphasis placed on spiritual practices and connecting with the divine, people of Hindu Indian ethnicity have strong third eye and crown chakras.

CHAPTER 11

Additional Chakras

The main purpose of this book is to provide detail about the seven most widely discussed chakras. The seven most widely discussed chakras are critical to understanding the other chakras because they are the building blocks to understanding other chakras. There are approximately 78,000 chakras being discussed at this time and there are many theories and representations used to discuss them. Some researchers, authors, healers, and teachers discuss additional chakras; while others discuss additional characteristics of the basic seven chakras or discuss chakras based on the fields of energy in which the chakras reside.

This section provides some additional evidence that I discovered during my research and use in my spiritual practice. Additional chakras can be found throughout the physical body and in the environment external to the person. This chapter includes discussion of some additional chakras. It is important to keep in mind this chapter does not address all chakras.

Other Chakras

We have discussed the seven major chakras in the human body in detail. We have also discussed that there many other chakras that are so many and so vast that discussing them all would be much to comprehensive for this text; however, there are some used often and are so beneficial to balance that presenting them in this text is important. Some people consider discussions about major chakras in addition to the seven major chakras discussed throughout this text as a new age approach; however, additional chakras have been used in Shamanic and Eastern spiritual and healing practices for hundreds of years.

Twelve Chakra System

Many interpretations of complete chakra systems exist. As previously mentioned, there are approximately 72,000 to 78,000 chakras in the human body. One of the most commonly discussed chakra systems is the twelve chakra system. Many variations of the 12 chakra system exist; Table 3 illustrates a combination of some of these approaches. The 12 chakra system includes the seven major chakras and the eighth, ninth, tenth, eleventh, and twelfth chakras. The 12 chakra system illustrates more fully how we connect to everything around us and how everything around us is connected to us.

Table 3. *Twelve Chakra Chart*

Chakra	Location	Also Known As	Purpose / Lesson
Twelfth	Surrounds the eleventh chakra	Divine Gateway	Universal Unity
Eleventh	Surrounds the body	Galactic	Mind Over Matter
Ninth	One and one-half feet above the head	Spirit	Seat of the Soul
Eighth	Just above the head	Soul Star	Transcend time to connect to spirit
Seventh	Top of the head	Crown	Connecting to universal law
Sixth	Forehead	Third Eye	Ability to see the truth
Fifth	Throat	Throat	Ability to speak the truth
Fourth	Center of chest	Heart	Self-love and love from and of others
Third	Epigastric area	Solar Plexus	Control of emotions
Second	Pelvis	Sacral	Flow of energy
First	Base of spine	Root	Grounding
Tenth	One and one half feet below the feet	Earth Star	Direct link to the energy of the earth

The Higher Chakras

Four additional, commonly discussed, chakras reside above the crown chakra and one additional commonly discussed, chakra resides below the root chakra. Collectively, the four of the additional chakras are known as the *Higher Chakras*. The higher chakras engage interaction between man and the chakras with the highest vibrations. An introduction to the higher chakras includes additional detail below.

The eighth and ninth chakras are located above the head. The eight chakra is located just above the head. The color of the eight chakra is either black or silver. Physically, it links to the thymus gland. The ninth chakra is located approximately one and a half feet above the head. The color of the ninth chakra is gold. Physically, it is connected to the diaphragm. The eighth chakra holds divine love, spiritual selflessness, and compassion. The eight chakra holds the Akashic Records, the Shadow Records, and the Book of Life. Together, the Akashic Records, the Shadow Records, and the Book of Life provide information about everything we have ever done and seen including any regrets that impact our present lives (Dale, 2016). The Akashic Records hold events, thoughts, and emotions that have occurred in the past, present, and future of a person's life time. The Shadow Records hold the events and behaviors of the shadow self that have occurred in the past, present, and future of a person's life time. The Book of Life mentioned here refers to an individual's chapter in the grand Book of Life that holds information about everything that has ever occurred across life times. The eighth chakra also holds information about life purpose and soul contract. Because the eighth chakra holds so much information, the eighth chakra is sometimes called the seat of the soul. The ninth chakra is where spiritual genetics reside. The ninth chakra reflects our purpose as defined by our soul. Together, the eighth and ninth chakras, make up the space where we interact with the universal source of all things. The eight chakra is where the source of everything lives within us. The ninth chakra is where we dwell within the source of everything.

Eleventh Chakra and Twelfth Chakras

The eleventh chakra and twelfth chakra surround the body. The eleventh chakra is closest to the body and is surrounded by the twelfth chakra. The color of the eleventh chakra is rose. Physically, the eleventh chakra connects to our connective tissue (Dale, 2016). The twelfth chakra is gold at the top and clear as it wraps around the entirety of the eleventh chakra and physical body. The twelfth chakra does not connect to any physical body part; rather, it acts as our spiritual skin (Dale, 2016). The twelfth chakra originates approximately one foot above a person's head and is also known as the *Soul Star*. Whereas, the eleventh chakra allows one to work with physical and supernatural powers when one desires to do so; the twelfth chakra allows one to connect to universal oneness. Together, the eleventh and twelfth chakras allow a person to experience true free will and to focus on the greatest good for all.

GROUNDING CHAKRAS

Tenth Chakra

The tenth chakra is located approximately one and one-half feet below the feet. The color of the tenth chakra is an earthy brown. Physically, this chakra connects to the center of our bones (Dale, 2016). The tenth chakra is our link to the world; to the energy of the earth. Additionally, the tenth chakra connects to ancestral inheritance and genetics. Through this chakra we are able to become aware of and receive the healing energies that exist in the natural world; the healing energies that spring forth from the earth.

Earth Star Chakra

The earth star chakra is located in the souls of the feet. It grounds a person's light / energy body to the center of the earth. The effect of a healthy earth star chakra is grounding into everyday reality. Being grounded into everyday reality removes feelings of unsteadiness and fear. Feelings of empowerment come from the connection between the earth star chakra and the center of the earth.

Hands and Feet

In addition to the seven major chakras previously discussed, chakras can be found in arms, hands, and feet. Chakras in the hand are located in the palms and the fingertips. Charkas in the palms of the hand run from front to back through the center of the palms of the hand. Palm chakras are often used to give massages, for feeling auras, and when giving Reiki and other healing treatments. Each fingertip has a chakra. Fingertip chakras are useful with pendulum and other divination techniques that require the use of your hands. Finger chakras are also helpful when giving massages or any type of hands on healing technique. Some healers use the chakras in the arms and hands in conjunction to direct energy toward the person who they are giving the healing treatment. Feet have two feeder chakras that receive from the earth. Grounding, connecting to the energy that comes from the earth, is what happens when these feeder chakras receive the earths energy and projects the energy upward. Energy received from the earth through the chakras in the feet are directed to the root chakra automatically. The receipt of earth energy impacts feelings of basic survival. Standing barefoot in grass can assist with grounding via the feeder chakras in the feet.

SPECIAL CHAKRAS

Past Life Chakra

The past life chakra is sometimes called the causal chakra. The past life chakra is approximately three finger breadths behind your ears;, just above the bony ridge on the side of your head. Although discussion of past life experiences are taboo for some and rejected by others, past life is just as important if not more important than the shadow self. Past life experiences have emotions tied to them that can impact present life. People with imbalances in their past life chakra appear stuck in the history. They are often fixated on things that went on decades and even centuries before they were born into this lifetime. The frequently bring up historical events in a way that shows they have trouble moving on from the event and / or the impact of the event. The past life chakra may be linked to a person's way of dealing with things or ancestral past life patterns that have been passed down for generations. People with imbalances past life chakras appear either dependent or self-directed. Meditating with a golden healer quartz crystal can help with healing the past life chakra.

Spleen Chakra

The spleen chakra is located near the spleen in the abdominal cavity. Imbalances in the spleen chakra tend to show themselves physically as immune problems and fatigue. Emotionally people with imbalanced spleen chakras tend to seem easily irritated or angry most of the time. For people with imbalanced spleen chakras, when the anger or irritation reaches a high level and fight or flight kicks in, the body begins to fight itself which leads to exhaustion of the physical body. People with blown open spleen chakras can rob others around them of energy as they continue on their self-destructive mission. In contrast, a person with a balanced spleen chakra appears self-assertive and empowered. People with balanced spleen chakras are natural born leaders; commonly classified as charismatic or transformational leaders because people easily follow their words and actions.

Color Associations

Each of the major chakras and some of the ones mentioned earlier in this chapter are specific colors. For example, the heart chakra is pink on one side and green on the other and the root chakra is red. Over time, people learned the connection between colors and manifesting the outcome they desire with and without intentionally working with chakras. Color associations can be found in what people wear and how people decorate. Color associations are often used to manifest ones desires or to present a specific picture. Common color associations include pink for self-love, orange for energy and passion, and red for setting boundaries and to show power. The color blue is often used to convey rational thinking and intellectual power. Purple conveys spirituality or royalty. A persons favorite colors are most likely the result of chakras that a person, over time and perhaps lifetimes, is familiar with. Favorite colors are colors that produce a specific feeling when seen or worn. Working with color associations requires paying attention to the colors that a person is drawn to and circumstances or situations surrounding when a person is drawn to the color(s). There as times when a person may subconsciously gravitate to the colors that we wear. This subconscious gravitation is the result of a metaphysical need that relates to specific chakras that your subconscious mind and / or spirit is working with. An example of this is wearing a blue suit to an interview; an interview is where a person needs to verbalize their truth in a way that sells his or her authentic self.

Conclusion

The purpose of this book was to discuss the seven major chakras. While writing this book, I discovered that simply discussing the seven major chakras only touched the surface and did not supply enough information for people to be able to heal themselves. Through the use of peer reviewed literature over many years and by using various complimentary healing modalities, I see how important understanding the subtle energy that resides in all of us it so true healing and to symptom management. With multiple certifications and diplomas, I assist myself, family, friends, and clients in the art and science of energy healing. I have now brought some of this knowledge to you. Understanding chakras helps us recognize the connection between the conscious physical body and the environment. Understanding chakras and how to harness the energy of the chakra system provides one with the ability to understand self and others. Awareness and understanding of the subtle energy system that resides in every one of us allows the ability to be truly free, be at one with everyone and everything, and live more comfortable lives. Harnessing the energy that is shared via the chakra system can help us live happy, productive, healthy and meaningful lives . . . *Harness the Inner You.*

Bibliography

Chakra Healing. (2016a). *All about the chakras: Awaken the chakras with these 12 powerful sound mantras.* Retrieved from http://www.chakrahealing.com/awaken-the-chakras-with-these-12-powerful-sound-mantras/

Chakra Healing. (2016b). *All about the seven chakras.* Retrieved from http://www.chakrahealing.com/awaken-the-chakras-with-these-12-powerful-sound-mantras/

Covington. C. (2018). *Plant alchemy: 22 essential oils for activating, opening and balancing the chakras.* Retrieved from https://www.consciouslifestylemag.com/22-essential-oils-for-chakras/

Crowhurst, M. (2017). *Chakra healing on demand: A quick course using micro meditations to heal.* Melbourne, Australia: Natural Healer.

Dale, C., & Wehrman, R. (2017). *The subtle body coloring book: Learning energetic anatomy from the chakras to the meridians and more.* Boulder, CO: Sounds True Publishing.

Dale, C. (2016). *Llwewllyn's complete book of chakras: Your definitive source of energy center knowledge for health, happiness, and spiritual Evolution.* St. Paul, MN: Llewellyn Publications.

Eason, C. (2018). *A little bit of auras.* New York, NY: Sterling Publishing.

Fenton, S. (2017). *Chakras plain and simple.* New York, NY: Sterling Publishing.

Ford, B. (2017). Cellular intelligence: Microphenomenology and the realities of being. *Progress in Biophysics and Molecular Biology, 131, 273-287.* http://dx.doi.org/10.1016/j.pbiomolbio.2017.08.012 0079-6107

Heymsfield, S., Burgeois, B., & Thomas, D. (2017). Assessment of human energy exchange: Historical overview. *European Journal of Clinical Nutrition, 71*, 294-300. http://dx.doi.org/10.1038/ejc.2016.221

Ar Yoga. (2011). Bija mantras the sounds of chakras: LAM, vam, ram, yam, ham, om. Retrieved from http://ar-yoga.com/2011/10/bija-mantras-the-sounds-of-the-chakras-lam-vam-ram-yam-ham-om/

Joshi, V. (2016). A quantum mechanical approach to study consciousness and healing. *International Journal of Scientific Research in Science and Technology, 2*(3), 181-184. Retrieved from http://ijsrst.com/

Jung, C. (1969). *Archetypes and the collective unconscious.* Princeton, NJ: Princeton University Press.

Kineman, J. (2017). A causal framework for integrating contemporary and Vedic holism. *Progress in Biophysics and Molecular Biology, 131, 402-423.* http://dx.doi.org/10.1016/j.biomolbio.2017.09.0110079-6107

Lefebvre, V. (2017). Theoretical modeling of the subject: Western and Eastern types of human reflexion. *Progress in Biophysics and Molecular Biology, 131*, 325-335. https://dx.doi.org/10.1016/j.pbiomolbio.2017.06.006

Leigh, A., & Mercree, C. (2016). *A little bit of chakras: An introduction to energy healing.* New York, NY: Sterling Publishing.

Matsuno, K. (2017). From quantum measurement to biology via retrocausality. *Progress in Biophysics and Molecular Biology, 131, 131-140.* https://dx.doi.org/10.1016/j.pbiomolbio.2017.06.012

Nayak B. S., Kumar, N., Aithal P., Shetty, S., Sirasanagandla, S., & Guru, A. (2015). Possibly active persistent thymus found in a human cadaver-A morphological study. *Online Journal of Health and Allied Sciences, 14*(4). Retrieved from https://www.researchgate.net/profile/Satheesha_B/publication/299563540_Possibly_Active_Persistent_Thymus_Found_in_a_Human_Adult_Cadaver_-A_Morphohistological_Study/links/56ff8d3808ae1408e15dc3e0/Possibly-Active-Persistent-Thymus-Found-in-a-Human-Adult-Cadaver-A-Morphohistological-Study.pdf

Rajagopal, R., Jois, S,. Majgi, S., Kumar, M., & Shashidher, H. (2018). Amelioration of mild and moderate depression through Pranic Healing as adjuvant therapy: Randomized double-blind controlled trial. *Australisian Psychiatry, 26*(1), 82-87. https://dx.doi.org/10.1177/1039856217726449

Sarma, D. (1961). *The Upanishads: An anthology.* Chaupatty: Bombay India: Bhavan's Book University.

Stephenson, J. (2017). What does energy mean?: An interdisciplinary conversation. *Energy Research & Social Science, 26,* 103-106. https://dx.doi.org/10.1016/j.erss.2017.01.014

Wauters, A. (1997). *Chakras and their archetypes uniting energy: Awareness and spiritual growth.* New York, NY: Crossing Press.

About the Author

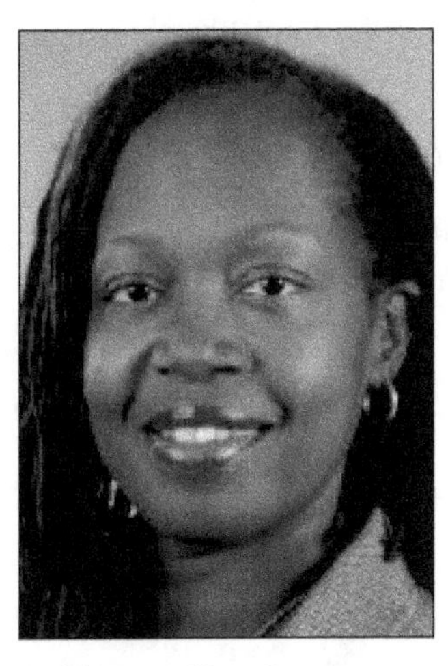

Dr. Temeaka Gray El is an Advanced Practice Registered Nurse with a Doctorate in Health and Wellness Psychology. Dr. G, as she is affectionally called by some of her students, patients, and clients, is the owner of Epiphany Consulting & Associates, LLC. and an Assistant Professor at the University of Toledo College of Nursing. Additionally, she is a Usui Ryoho Reiki Master, who is also trained in Karuna Ki and Kundalini Reiki. She is also skilled in the use of Quantum Touch as a healing modality and holds diplomas in Crystal Healing and Energy Healing. As part of her holistic practice, she teaches meditation techniques and assists her clients with raising their subtle body energy frequencies, so they can help create an environment of mind, body, and spiritual peace. Her goal is to bring healing to create harmony in the world through the use of energy healing techniques.

Contact Information

Website: https://temeakagray.wixsite.com/epiphanyconsulting

Email: Temeaka.gray@gmail.com

Phone: (419)464-8875

Facebook

https://www.facebook.com/temeaka.gray

https://www.facebook.com/Calm-Wolf-Running-1021658894655429/

https://www.facebook.com/Epiphany-Health-Tips-289518337764385/

Twitter: @DocGrayCNP

www.ingramcontent.com/pod-product-compliance
Lightning Source LLC
LaVergne TN
LVHW020653100826
845148LV00012B/2475

* 9 7 8 1 7 3 5 6 8 1 7 7 1 *